NRF2 as a

Heba Kamal Nabih

NRF2 as a Central Point in Cancer Metastasis

LAP LAMBERT Academic Publishing

Table of contents

- ### What is NRF2?

Nrf2, a basic leucine zipper (bZIP) transcription factor, is a member of the Cap-N-Collar family of regulatory proteins that includes NF-E2, Nrf1, Nrf3, Bach1, and Bach2 **(Motohashi et al., 2002).** The gene encoding for 605 amino acids of NRF2 is localized in chromosome 2q31 within a 2.2 kb transcript and comprises six exons **(Venugopal and Jaiswal, 1996; Hooijberg et al., 1999).** Based on numerous studies, Nrf2, initially recognized as a key transcription factor of various antioxidant and cytoprotective enzymes, possibly plays important roles during the progression of human tumor **(Figure 1) (Long et al., 2000; Chen and Kunsch, 2004; Lee and Surh, 2005).**

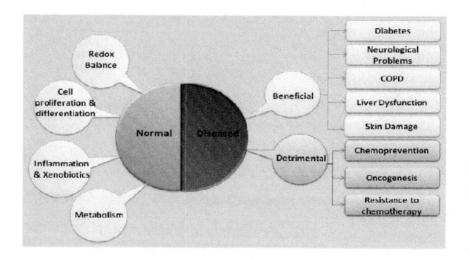

Fig.1: Functions of Nrf2. Nrf2 maintains homeostasis in the body. It plays a beneficial role in several diseased conditions, but during cancer, it plays a detrimental role in promoting cancer progression.

- ## The critical role of NRF2 in cancer

Accumulating evidence suggests that the activation of NRF2 is critical for tumor cell proliferation, growth, and survival **(Jia *et al.*, 2016)**. Moreover, NRF2 activation is thought to be the main cause of resistance to chemotherapy and radiotherapy **(Figure 2) (Choi and Kwak, 2016)**.

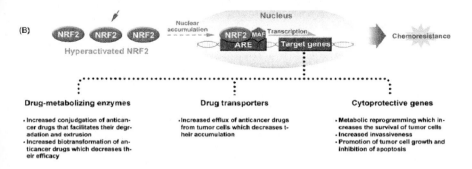

Fig. 2: The hyperactivation process of NRF2.

Nrf2 is responsible for regulation of expression of efflux transporters especially from ATP-binding cassette (ABC) family which pumps out xenobiotics from the cell against a concentration gradient. Nrf2 binds to the ARE-like sequences in the promoters of multidrug resistance-associated proteins (MRP) genes like Mrp1, Mrp2, Mrp3, Mrp4, and Abcg2 and enhances their expressions, thus confers chemo resistance in cells. Nrf2 plays key role in the development of drug resistance in patients undergoing chemotherapy. The activity of Nrf2 in cancer cells decreases their sensitivity to the common chemotherapeutic agents like doxorubicin, carboplatin, cisplatin, etc. RNAi-mediated inhibition of Nrf2 signaling has been documented to reverse drug resistance **(Lister *et al.*, 2011)**. Repression of Nrf2 promotes the cytotoxic effects of g-irradiation towards lung and pancreatic cancer cell lines. In vitro studies have revealed that Nrf2 signaling activity is downregulated in the doxorubicin- sensitive human ovarian carcinoma cell line, A2780 **(PÖlÖnen and Levonen, 2016)**.

- **Drug efflux transporters regulated by NRF2 in cancer**

MRPs

Multidrug resistance proteins (MRPs) belong to a group of membrane-anchored transporters that are well known to be responsible for the active transport of a wide range of compounds across biological membranes, including drugs through the binding and subsequent hydrolysis of ATP at their nucleotide-binding domains which provide energy for this active transport **(Chen *et al.*, 1999)**. GSH (glutathione) is essential for the efflux of certain compounds by interaction with MRPs **(Ballatori *et al.*, 2005)**. Several lines of evidence support that NRF2- dependent high expression level of MRPs involves in developmental chemoresistance in human tumor **(Duong *et al.*, 2014; Mahaffey *et al.*, 2009, 2012; Sasaki *et al.*, 2012; Vollrath *et al.*, 2006; Xu *et al.*, 2014)**. By measuring GSH levels, they found that MRP1 protects tumor cells from the toxic effects of xenobiotics through the co-transport of GSH and the xenobiotic from the intracellular compartment to the extracellular medium. These findings demonstrated that MRP exerts effect in drug detoxification. In human ovarian cancer, doxorubicin was found to induce 1.6-fold expression of MRP1 through activating NRF2 compared with normal cells. This abnormal expression of MRP1 accelerates the extrusion of doxorubicin and results in approximately two-fold reduction on its cytotoxicity **(Shim *et al.*, 2009)**, and similar results were also found in leukemia **(Xu *et al.*, 2014)** and NSCLC (Non-Small-Cell Lung Carcinoma) cells **(Young *et al.*, 2001)**. Although several anticancer drugs have been found to be transported by MRP4/ABCC4, the role of MRP4 in cancers or chemotherapy is still plausible and not fully understood. The increased MRP4 expression could be ascribed to NRF2 activation, but whether MRP4 reduces accumulation of these drugs inside cells or it is only a part of results of NRF2 activation needs further confirmations

(Huang and Sadee, 2006). MRP5 is highly expressed in neuroglioma (16-fold) compared with normal tissues. Treatment with NRF2 inhibitors (chrysin and apigenin) could decrease the level of MRP5 by two-fold and increase the cytotoxicity of doxorubicin, indicating that MRP5 overexpression is NRF2-dependent. Long-term exposure to platinum drugs like cisplatin induces an approximately two-fold increase on MRP5 expression by up-regulating NRF2 in refractory lung cancer **(Oguri et al., 2000)**, further supporting the role of NRF2 in MRP5-induced chemoresistance.

BCRP

BCRP/ABCG2 (breast cancer resistance protein/ATP-binding cassette, subfamily G member 2) and was originally cloned from DRN-resistant MCF7 breast cancer cells. NRF2 interacts with the antioxidant response element (ARE) area in the promoter of BCRP and regulates its expression in human cells **(Singh et al., 2010)**, so in some tumor cells with high expression of NRF2, BCRP is usually maintained at high level (3–4-fold) compared with their parental cells **(Doyle and Ross, 2003; Ma and Wink, 2010; Maliepaard et al., 2001)**. Importantly, its abnormal up-regulation contributes to tumor resistance towards targeted cancer therapies. Clinically, a significant correlation between resistance to 5- Fluorouracil (5-FU) and expression level of BCRP has been found in 140 breast cancer tissue specimens **(Yuan et al., 2008)**, which is consistent with a previous study indicating that overexpressed BCRP leads to resistance by significantly increasing 5-FU efflux outside breast cancer MCF7 cells **(Robey et al., 2001)**.

- ■ **Cancers overexpressed NRF2**

Overexpression of Nrf2 has been found in many types of cancer cells including lung cancer **(Solis et al., 2010)**, endometrial carcinoma **(Chen et al., 2011)**, hepatocellular carcinoma **(Ma et al., 2011)**, ovarian cancer **(Konstantinopoulos et al., 2011)**, pancreatic cancer **(Lister et al., 2011)**, thyroid cancer **(Du et al., 2011)**, and gallbladder cancer (**Wang** *et al.,* **2010**). Enhanced cancer cell growth and survival result from the overexpression of nuclear Nrf2. In gallbladder cancer, significant correlations have been found between the high Nrf2 expression and the tumor differentiation, Nevin staging, metastasis, and shorter overall survival times. The data suggested that Nrf2 had the potential to serve as an independent prognostic factor in gallbladder cancer (**Wang** *et al.,* **2010**). In non–small cell lung carcinoma, the overexpression of nuclear Nrf2 was principally attributable to worse recurrence-free survival and overall survival in patients with squamous cell carcinoma who received platinum-based treatment, which suggested that Nrf2 activation played a role in chemotherapy resistance (**Solis** *et al.,* **2010**). Moreover, Nrf2 activation was confirmed again in patients with epithelial ovarian cancer who showed resistance to platinum-based chemotherapy (**Konstantinopoulos** *et al.,* **2011**). In fully malignant cells Nrf2 activity provides growth advantage by increasing cancer chemoresistance and enhancing tumor cell growth. Abundant Nrf2 protein causes increased expression of genes involved in drug metabolism thereby increasing the resistance to chemotherapeutic drugs and radiotherapy. In addition, high Nrf2 protein level is associated with poor prognosis in cancer (**Sporn and Liby, 2012**). In short, Nrf2 plays a key role in tumor progression and serves to determine clinical responses to chemotherapy.

- ▪ **The Dual role of NRF2 in cancer**

The prognosis of patients with tumors expressing high levels of Nrf2 is poor partly due to Nrf2's ability to increase cancer cell proliferation and promote chemoresistance and radioresistance (**Zhang** *et al.,* **2015**). NRF2 target genes regulate redox homeostasis, drug metabolism and excretion, energetic metabolism, iron metabolism, amino acid metabolism, survival, proliferation, autophagy, proteasomal degradation, DNA repair, and mitochondrial physiology (**Hayes and Dinkova-Kostova, 2014; Lee** *et al.,* **2017**). In the last decade, many studies have described that NRF2 activation in cancer cells promotes cancer progression (**DeNicola** *et al.*, **2011; Satoh** *et al.*, **2013; Tao** *et al.*, **2017b**) and metastasis (**Wang** *et al.*, **2016**), and also confers resistance to chemo and radiotherapy (**Padmanabhan** *et al.*, **2006; Singh** *et al.*, **2006**) (**Figure 3**).

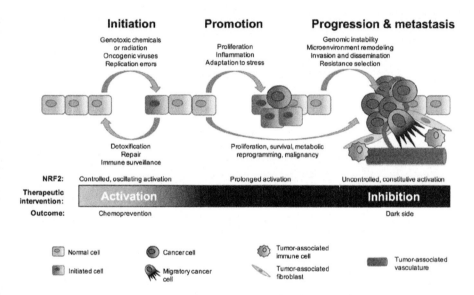

Fig.3: Dual Roles of NRF2 in Cancer. The modes of NRF2 regulation during the multistep development of cancer determine its functional outcome and influence the therapeutic intervention that could be used. Controlled activation of NRF2 in normal cells via the canonical mechanism prevents cancer initiation and is suitable for cancer chemoprevention strategies. Prolonged (non-canonical) or constitutive (loss of regulatory mechanisms) activation of NRF2 participates in cancer promotion, progression, and metastasis. This dark side can be antagonized by inhibition of NRF2.

- **NRF2 and angiogenesis**

Angiogenesis is the formation of new blood vessels from an existing vascular bed (**Folkman and Shing, 1992**). The hypothesis that a tumor depends on active angiogenesis was first proposed by Folkman in 1971 (**Hillen and Griffioen, 2007**).

Nrf2 is essential for the normal endothelial angiogenic processes through preserving a normal endothelial phenotype and vascular integrity **(Bailey-Downs *et al.*, 2012; Valcarcel-Ares *et al.*, 2012)**. It is possible that the role of Nrf2 in the tumor angiogenic processes may be to affect the biological behavior of intratumoral endothelial cells. Reactive oxygen species (ROS) are also important stimuli for angiogenic signaling **(North *et al.*, 2005) (Figure 4)**.

- ## The role of ROS in cancer incidence

Cancer is one of the leading cause of death worldwide; in2012 about 14.1 million new incidence of cancer and 8.2 million cancer related deaths occurred globally according to WHO **(WHO, 2014)**. Oxidative stress is one of crucial causes responsible for cancer. There are many intrinsic factors generated during metabolic and pathological processes, which include reactive oxygen species (ROS) resulting in oxidative stress. It occurs when there is an imbalance in a cell between the pro-oxidant species that can damage key macromolecules, and the anti-oxidative mechanisms that have evolved to protect the body from these potentially harmful species **(Jaiswal, 2004)**. Radical species have a single unpaired electronand can cause damage to proteins, lipids and DNA, resulting in reduced function leading to malignancy **(Breimer, 1990) (Figure 5)**.

- ## Targets of NRF2 signaling

One of the best studied Nrf2 target genes is HO-1, a member of the heme oxygenase family **(Lavrovsky *et al.*, 1994)**. In cancer, increased expression of HO-1 is correlated with decreased overall survival in non-small cell lung cancer **(Tsai *et al.*, 2012)**, and it is highly expressed in castration-resistant prostate cancer **(Li *et al.*, 2011)**. It may also reduce the immune response, as HO-1 directly interacts with

STAT3 **(Degradation *et al.*, 2012)**. The role of HO-1 in angiogenesis is well established. HO-1 has been recognized as a proangiogenic enzyme. The induction of HO-1 by hemin results in corresponding elevation in vascular endothelial growth factor (VEGF) production **(Jozkowicz *et al.*, 2003; Li *et al.*, 2005; Meng *et al.*, 2010)**. VEGF promotes proliferation, sprouting, migration, and tube formation of endothelial cells, VEGF is well recognized as an essential regulator of tumor angiogenesis **(Ferrara *et al.*, 2003; Hicklin and Ellis, 2005)**. VEGF increased vascular permeability, resulting in the accumulation of extracellular matrix proteins, such as fibrinogen and vitronectin. These proteins induced the proliferation and migration of endothelial cells and promoted the formation of new blood vessels. VEGF activated Nrf2-ARE signal pathway in an ERK1/2-depentent manner. In one *in vitro* study, primary BMECs (Brain Microvascular Endothelial Cells) were incubated with VEGF, and the Nrf2-ARE system was evaluated by Western blot analysis. The results indicated that VEGF may activate the Nrf2-ARE signal in a dose- and time-dependent manner via the ERK1/2 signaling pathway **(Liwen *et al.*, 2016)**.

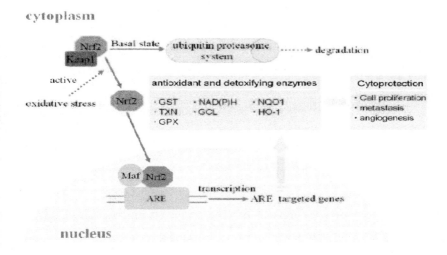

Fig. 4: The Nrf2 signal under oxidative stress. Normally, Nrf2 as an inactive complex remains in the cytosol by binding to Keap1 and is targeted for proteasomal degradation. Under oxidative stress, Nrf2 dissociates from Keap1 and translocates into the nucleus to form a heterodimer with small Maf proteins and subsequently binds to the antioxidant response element (ARE), leading to antioxidant and cytoprotection. GCL, glutamylcysteine ligase; GST, glutathione S-transferases; GPX, glutathione peroxidase; HO-1, heme oxygenase-1; NAD(P)H, nicotinamide adenine dinucleotide phosphate; NQO1, nicotinamide adenine dinucleotide phosphate quinone oxidoreductase 1; TXN, thioredoxin.

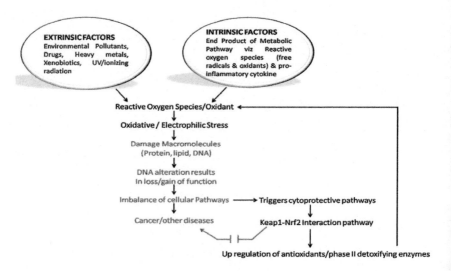

Fig. 5: Flow diagram showing factors involved in ROS generation and cascade of events in detoxification.

HO-1 was found in vascular smooth muscle cells **(Duckers *et al.*, 2001; Dulak *et al.*, 2002)**, keratinocytes **(Jazwa *et al.*, 2006)**, macrophages, and tumor cells **(Dulak *et al.*, 2008)**. The action of Nrf2 in tumor angiogenesis may occur through the HO-1–driven VEGF pathway **(Figure 6)**. HO-1 is a downstream target of stromal cell-derived factor 1 in endothelial cells, and it promotes angiogenesis in a VEGF-independent fashion. In a mouse xenograft model, not only did HO-1 inhibition decrease microvessel density, but it also decreased VEGF and HIF-1α levels. High HO-1 has also been associated with increased microvessel density in bladder tumors **(Miyake et al., 2011)**. HO-1 may also activate extrinsic mechanisms of metastasis in the tumor microenvironment, as the expression of HO-1 was found to be increased in metastatic prostate tumors **(Nemeth et al., 2015)**.

HO-1 is an NRF2-regulated stress response protein that catalyzes the catabolism of the prooxidant heme to carbon monoxide (CO), biliverdin and free iron **(Mayerhofer et al., 2004)**. It has important cellular functions in growth regulation and self-defense processes resisting a wide range of external stress stimuli. An increasing number of studies supporting the pivotal role of Nrf2 in angiogenesis show that Nrf2 may promote vascular development via protection of retina from hyperoxia-induced oxidative stress **(Uno et al., 2010)**; these studies also indicate that Nrf2 blockade suppresses tumor cell angiogenesis and migration *in vivo* and *in vitro*. These results suggest that Nrf2 can regulate angiogenesis via HO-1 mediated HIF-1α /VEGF signaling pathways **(Kim et al., 2011; Ji et al., 2013; Ji et al., 2014) (Figure 7)**.

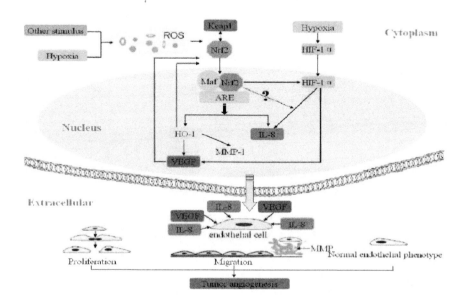

Fig. 6: The possible pathways of Nrf2 in tumor angiogenesis. Hypoxia induces Nrf2 by production of reactive oxygen species (ROS), leading to the up-regulation of the expression of HO-1 and IL-8. In turn, over-expression of heme oxygenase-1 (HO-1) triggers the production of vascular endothelial growth factor (VEGF), and VEGF up-regulation will activate Nrf2, resulting in augmentation of this feedback. In addition, Nrf2-induced VEGF production is regulated by hypoxia-inducible factor (HIF)-1α. Moreover, Nrf2 may affect tumor angiogenesis by participating the regulation of HIF-1α on interleukin-8 (IL-8). Finally, the proangiogenic factors affect the biologic behavior of endothelial cells, including promotion of proliferation, migration, and formation of capillary-like structures and reduction of adhesion to extracellular matrix proteins, all of which contribute to tumor angiogenesis. ARE, antioxidant response element; and MMP, matrix metalloproteinase.

Overexpression of HO-1 has been found in chemoresistant myeloma **(Nowis et al., 2008)**, lung cancer **(Jeon et al., 2012)**, myeloid leukemia **(Heasman et al., 2011)**. In a mouse model, HO-1 overexpression in macrophages accelerated angiogenic potential of human pancreatic cancer MiaPaca2 cells, and this is closely associated with promoted local tumor growth. By enhancing cell proliferation and improving resistance to oxidative stress and apoptotic stimuli induced by chemotherapies, HO-1 may play a critical role in developed chemoresistance.

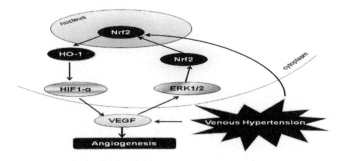

Fig.7: The proposed signaling pathway of this study: Venous Hypertension may participate in angiogenesis via activating Nrf2-ARE and HIF-1α/VEGF signaling pathway in AVMs. *In vitro*, we observed that there existed a VEGF/Nrf2 positive feed back loop in mice BMECs. VEGF activated Nrf2-ARE system via ERK1/2 signaling pathway, in turn, upregulated the expression of itself.

Besides, Nrf2 palys a crucial role in the process of angiogenesis and the activator of Nrf2 t-BHQ may also upregulate VEGF expression via Nrf2/HO-1/HIF-1α pathways. Furthermore, knockout of Nrf2 impairs VEGF-induced BMECs migration and angiogenesis *ex vivo*.

- **Invasion and metastasis of cancer**

Invasion of local tissue is the direct result of tumor growth. As a tumor grows, nutrients are provided by direct diffusion from the general circulation and from the tumor's own vascular supply. Tumor cells are continuously being shed into the venous and lymphatic circulation spawning independent tumor nodules, metastases. Metastasis is a highly complicated phenomenon requiring the interaction of many different types of cells, connective tissues and blood vessel components within different organs. The complex metastasis process is the leading cause of cancer-related deaths. Reinforcing the understanding of the underlying mechanisms could be conducive to facilitating the development of effective metastasis-targeted therapies and improving the overall prognosis. The presence of malignant cells in the circulation does not necessarily mean that metastasis will result. For most tumors, the neoplastic population must expand considerably before invasion and metastasis can occur. This expansion may be clonal and limited to a more aggressive subpopulation of neoplastic cells, and resistant to conventional chemotherapy or radiotherapy **(Figure 8) (Arguello *et al.*, 1991; Chan and Wang, 2015)**.

- **Hallmark of hypoxia**

The importance of the tumor microenvironment for cancer progression and therapeutic resistance is an emerging focus of cancer biology. Hypoxia, or low oxygen, is a hallmark of solid tumors that promotes metastasis and represents a significant obstacle to successful cancer therapy. Hypoxia-inducible factor 1 (HIF-1) is considered the main effecter of the cellular response to hypoxia, stimulating the transcription of genes involved in promoting angiogenesis and altering cellular metabolism **(Toth and Warfel, 2017)**.

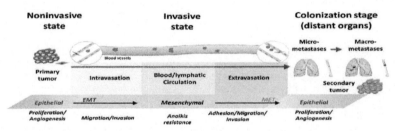

Fig. 8: The schematic of cancer metastasis: From primary site to disseminated organs.

The main regulator of the cellular hypoxic response is the HIF-1 transcription factor. In the presence of low oxygen, HIF-α accumulates and translocates into the nucleus where it activates genes containing a hypoxia response element **(GÖrlach, 2014)**. Many HIF-1 target genes are pro-angiogenic factors, such as VEGF **(Krock et al., 2011)**. These factors stimulate the growth of neovessels, rescuing tumor cells from their hypoxic state and promoting tumor progression. In addition, the expression of a hypoxic gene signature has been demonstrated to correlate with increased metastasis, changes in cellular metabolism, and chemoresistance **(Rankin and Giaccia, 2016)**. In recent years, it has become evident that ROS also serve as a signaling mechanism for low levels of cellular oxygen. Increased ROS promote the nuclear localization of NF-kB (nuclear factor kappa-light-chain-enhancer of activated B cells), which increases the transcription of HIF1A and its downstream targets **(Bonello et al., 2007)**. HIF-1 has been described as a key regulator of the inflammatory response and immune cell function **(Palazon et al., 2014)**. Another important mechanism by which hypoxia causes chemoresistance is by increasing the expression of transporters, particularly the multidrug resistance protein (MDR-1). The expression of HIF-1 and MDR-1 is significantly correlated in colorectal and gastric cancer tissues **(Liu et al., 2008; Ding et al., 2010; Danza et al., 2016)**.

Moreover, bladder cancer tissues resistant to cisplatin treatment had higher levels of both of these proteins, and in vitro studies in bladder cancer cell lines demonstrated that increased HIF-1α levels enhanced MDR-1 expression and promoted cisplatin resistance **(Sun *et al.*, 2016)**. A similar phenomenon has also been described in pancreatic cancer. In this case, a different ABC family member, ABCG2, was correlated with HIF-1α expression. This family member is a direct target of HIF-1, and promotes resistance to gemcitabine in pancreatic cancer cells **(He *et al.*, 2016)**. In addition, a separate study by Syu et al. suggested that Nrf2 is involved in drug transporter-mediated chemoresistance in hypoxia. Because Nrf2 can also activate other ABC family transporters, it is possible that the HIF-1 and Nrf2 pathways interact to promote resistance to chemotherapy, particularly within the hypoxic tumor microenvironment. Although HIF-1 and Nrf2 signaling are both regulated by the presence of reactive oxygen, there is evidence that these two signaling pathways are interacting to promote metastasis and play complementary roles in chemoresistance **(Syu *et al.*, 2016) (Figure 9)**.

- **The hero side of NRF2**

In the absence of oxidative stress, Nrf2 is bound by its negative regulator, KEAP1 (Kelch-like erythroid cell-derived protein with cap'n'collar [CNC] homology-associated protein 1). Binding to KEAP1 promotes the ubiquitination of Nrf2 by Cullin3 and facilitates its subsequent degradation by the 26S proteasome **(Bryan *et al.*, 2013)**. This interaction is abrogated by the presence of oxidative stress, as KEAP1 is oxidized on several key cysteine residues, which alters its conformation and allows Nrf2 to escape ubiquitination-mediated degradation and translocate into the nucleus, where it binds to promoters containing ARE. Activation of Nrf2 promotes the transcription of Several Phase II detoxification enzymes such as glutathione-S transferases(GSTs), NADP (H): quinine oxidoreductase (NQO1), glutathione per-oxidases (GPx), catalase, superoxide dismutases (SODs), epoxidehydrolase, heme oxygenase (HO1), UDP-glucuronosyl transferases(UGTs), and gamma-glutamylcysteine synthetase (GCL) **(Lee et al., 2009)**, in a single word Nrf2 serves as a hero which reduce the levels of damaging ROS in the cell, thus maintaining homeostasis **(Gorrini et al., 2013)**. Oh et al. recently discovered that NQO1 expression increases the half-life of HIF-1α protein, and overexpression of NQO1 is sufficient to stabilize HIF-1α levels in normoxia. And overexpression of NQO1 increases the level of HIF-1α. Nrf2 target genes to increase HIF-1 signaling could contribute to the finding that NQO1 is a negative prognosticator for 5-year survival in colon cancer **(Oh et al., 2016).** Moreover, HIF-1 signaling and pro-angiogenic factors have been shown to increase Nrf2 activation **(Li et al., 2016)**. Loboda et al. found that, in endothelial cells, HIF-1α stabilization repressed Nrf2 signaling through a Bach1-dependent mechanism **(Loboda et al., 2009)**. In a separate study, treatment with the natural product andrographolide, an Nrf2 inducer **(Guan et al., 2013)**, decreased HIF-1α expression. Suggesting that this molecule activates Nrf2 signaling to actively block signaling by HIF-1 **(Lin et al., 2017)**. Taken together, these studies indicate that the HIF-1 and Nrf2 stress response pathways exist in a complex, interactive signaling network. Hypoxia poses a major problem for the treatment of solid tumors. In response to low oxygen, tumor cells activate a coordinated expression of genes that promote angiogenesis and metastasis, and therapeutic resistance. Growing evidence indicates that Nrf2 and HIF-1 signaling both contribute to the oncogenic phenotypes associated with hypoxia. Understanding the distinct and overlapping contributions of these signaling pathways is an exciting area of research, particularly in the context of the hypoxic tumor microenvironment. There have been successful attempts to target HIF-1 and Nrf2, and blocking these pathways synchronously has great potential for anti-cancer therapy. In the future, determining the molecular mechanisms by which the HIF-1 and Nrf2 signaling pathways communicate and compensate for each other will undoubtedly provide new targets to exploit oxidative stress in cancer and other disease states.

- **Drug-metabolizing enzymes regulated by NRF2 in cancer**

NQO1

NAD(P)H:quinone oxidoreductase 1 (NQO1) is a flavoenzyme belonging to NAD(P)H dehydrogenase family that catalyzes the transformation of quinones into hydroquinone via pyridine nucleotide cofactors NADH or NADPH **(Ross et al., 2000)**. NQO1 also scavenges superoxide to defend against oxidative stress induced by cytotoxic substances **(Benson et al., 1980; Lili Ji et al., 2014)**.

CYP1B1

CYP1B1 is a member of human cytochrome P450 (CYP) enzymes **(Hayes and Dinkova-Kostova, 2014)**. CYP1B1 mainly metabolizes 17 bestradiol and foreign chemicals including chemotherapeutic drugs, such as cyclophosphamide and taxanes, through hydroxylation **(Lewis, 2004; Nebert et al., 2013)**. By altering the structure of drug substrates, CYP1B1 may affect the tubulin- or DNA-binding activities of these drugs and decrease the sensitivity of cancer cells in reacting to anticancer agents.

GSTs

Glutathione S-transferases belong to a key superfamily of phase II metabolic enzymes. To date, a large part of them were reported to be positively regulated by NRF2 **(Hayes and Dinkova-Kostova, 2014)**. These enzymes catalyze the binding of electrophilic group of substrates to the sulfydryl on glutathione (GSH), thus facilitating the subsequent detoxification process coordinated with MRPs **(Hayes et al., 2005)**. The contribution of human GSTP1 in tumor tissues to chemoresistance has been confirmed. In breast cancer, high expression of GSTP1 is an unfavorable marker that causes more aggressive tumors with poorer prognosis than corresponding GSTP1-negative tumor **(Huang et al., 2003; Su et al., 2003)**. Noda et al. (2012)

investigated the effects of GSTP1 on patients with CRC during treatment with 5-FU or oxaliplatin, and they found that GSTP1-deficient patients have more positive response to these drugs, which highlights the predictive value of GSTP1 in chemotherapies. In resistant lung adenocarcinoma, GSTP1 is increased to about 1.5-fold and contributes to intrinsic resistance towards cisplatin **(Arai et al., 2008)**. MGSTs (microsomal glutathione transferases) are predominantly located in the endoplasmic reticulum and outer mitochondrial membrane. Researchers studying the association between MGST1 and doxorubicin **(Scotlandi et al., 2009)**, their results revealed that high expression of MGST1 is significantly associated with doxorubicin, melphalan and chlorambucil-resistance **(Johansson et al., 2007)**, and facilitating their conjugation with GSH. Transporters, especially MRP1 and MRP2, show higher transport velocities (Vmax values) for the exertion of GSH-conjugated drug, which decreases the concentration of them in cancer cells and results in acquired drug resistance **(Johansson et al., 2010)**.

ALDHs

Aldehyde dehydrogenases (ALDHs) belong to a superfamily of NAD(P)-dependent enzymes involved in oxidizing aldehydes of xenobiotics into their corresponding carboxylic acids. Recent studies indicated that drug-induced ALDHs could activate Notch1 and Shh signaling pathway to support tumor cell growth **(Nishikawa et al., 2013)**. ALDHs mediated the resistance to temozolomide in glioblastoma **(Schafer et al., 2012)**.

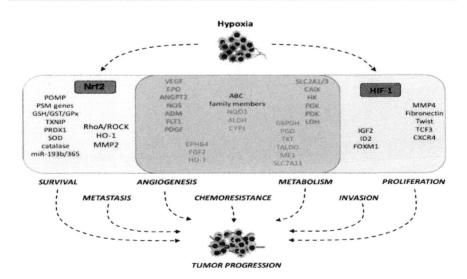

Fig. 9: Tumor hypoxia activates Nrf2 and HIF-1 signaling to promote tumor progression through the activation of distinct and overlapping pathways. Through their respective target genes, Nrf2 and HIF-1 activate redundant pathways to stimulate angiogenesis, chemoresistance, and metabolic shifts, as well as unique pathways that contribute to tumor progression, such as survival and metastasis (Nrf2) and invasion and proliferation (HIF-1). Blue box: Nrf2 target genes; red box: HIF-1 target genes. Genes within the purple box (blue text: Nrf2 targets; red text: HIF-1 targets) contribute to redundant pathways. Purple text indicates classes of genes regulated by both Nrf2 and HIF-1. Nrf2: nuclear factor, erythroid 2-like 2; HIF-1: hypoxia inducible factor 1; POMP: proteasome maturation protein; PSM: proteasome; GSH: glutathione; GST: glutathione S-transferase; GPx: glutathione peroxidase; TXNIP: thioredoxin interacting protein; PRDX1: peroxiredoxin 1; SOD: superoxide dismutase; miR: microRNA; RhoA: Ras homolog family member A; ROCK: RhoA kinase; HO-1: heme oxygenase 1; MMP: matrix metalloproteinase; VEGF: vascular endothelial growth factor; EPO: erythropoietin; ANGPT2: angiopoietin 2; NOS: nitric oxide synthase; ADM: adrenomedullin; FLT1: Fms-related tyrosine kinase 1; PDGF: platelet-derived growth factor; EPHB4: EPH receptor 4; FGF2: fibroblast growth factor 2; G6PDH: glucose-6-phosphate dehydrogenase; PGD: phosphogluconate dehydrogenase; TKT: transketolase; TALDO: transaldolase; ME1: malic enzyme 1; SLC: solute carrier family; ABC: ATP-binding cassette; NQO1: NADPH: quinone dehydrogenase 1; ALDH: aldehyde dehydrogenase; CYP: cytochrome p450; CAIX: carbonic anhydrase IX; HK: hexokinase; PGK: phosphoglycerate kinase;

PDK: pyruvate dehydrogenase kinase; LDH: lactate dehydrogenase; IGF2: insulin-like growth factor 2; ID2: inhibitor of DNA binding 2; FOXM1: forkhead box M1; TCF3: transcription factor 3; CXCR4: C-X-C motif chemokine receptor 4.

- ### P53 regulation by NRF2 expression

P53 is a tumor suppressor that also promotes an anti-oxidative stress metabolic program and glutaminolysis (a metabolic process that promotes the conversion of glutamine to glutamate that is often active in cancer cells) **(Rotblat *et al.*, 2012)**. An increase in the expression levels of Nrf2 could thereby increase the inhibition of p53, and unexpectedly ceases ROS based apoptotic signals, enhancing cellular survival leading to tumorigenesis **(Wakabayashi *et al.*, 2010)**. ROS are a byproduct of respiration and exposure to the environment **(Malinin *et al.*, 2011; Hwang and Lee, 2011)**. When in excess, ROS can damage DNA, proteins and lipids and promote mutations that may contribute to onset of a wide spectrum of human diseases particularly cancer **(Choi *et al.*, 2010)**. Nrf2 has also been shown to aid tumor cells resistance towards chemopreventive/chemotherapeutic agents, with one instance being Nrf2 regulating the expression of the multidrug resistant protein-3 (MRP3) in both human bronchial epithelial and NSCLC **(Mahaffey *et al.*, 2009)**. This protein when combined with an up regulation of detoxification enzymes, like GSTs, can lead to the increased hydrophilicity, and excretion of a variety of cytotoxic agents utilized in chemotherapy including chlorambucil, cisplatin, etoposide, and doxorubicin **(Meijerman *et al.*, 2008)**.

It is becoming more evident that, at the functional level, p53 and NRF2 play similar roles and are both providing cells with enhanced capacity to mitigate oxidative stress. Interestingly, recent findings from the Zhang lab indicate that p21, a p53 target gene **(El-Deiry *et al.*, 1993; Pang *et al.*, 2011)**, stabilizes NRF2 by binding to KEAP1 and interfering with its ability to promote NRF2 ubiquitylaton and proteasomal degradation **(Chen *et al.*, 2009)**. On the other hand, previous findings from the Shaul lab indicate that NQO1, an NRF2 target, interacts with p53 **(Asher *et al.*, 2005)** and blocks its degradation by the 20S proteasome **(Asher *et al.*, 2001)**, a degradation process that is independent of MDM2 and ubiquitin **(Asher *et al.*, 2002)**. These findings support the premise of an interesting cross talk between these two transcription factors and raise the question of whether there is a positive feedback loop between NRF2 and p53 and whether cancer cells enhance their resistance to oxidative stress by utilizing this putative positive feedback loop. Indeed, p53 deficient HCT116 colon carcinoma cells exhibited reduced induction of NRF2 target genes as compared with p53 proficient HCT116 cells following challenge with oxidative stress **(Kalo *et al.*, 2012)** suggesting that p53 may be important for NRF2 activation in cancer cells. However, this model may not be complete, as it was recently shown that *MDM2* is a transcriptional target of NRF2 through which NRF2 negatively regulates p53 **(You *et al.*, 2011)**. The relationship between NRF2 and p53 may well be dependent on the cellular and biological context. The cancer cells will utilize endogenous protective mechanisms to evolve chemoresistance **(Saxena *et al.*, 2011)**.

- **NRF2 and DNA damage**

NRF2 activation in non-transformed cells protects against DNA damaging agents and prevents carcinogenesis, as has been described in multiple studies **(Frohlich *et al.*, 2008; Singh *et al.*, 2012; Mathew *et al.*, 2014; Tao *et al.*, 2015; Das *et al.*, 2017; Jeayeng *et al.*, 2017)**, whereas constitutive activation of NRF2 protects cancer cells from genotoxic chemo- and radiotherapies, making them refractory to treatment **(Sekhar and Freeman, 2015; Jayakumar *et al.*, 2015)**. The DNA protective effects of NRF2 seem dependent on the expression of DNA damage response genes and not only on the antioxidant functions of NRF2 **(Jayakumar *et al.*, 2015)**. NRF2 also prevents DNA damage indirectly by reducing the amount of ROS, which in addition to generating oxidative DNA damage also cause abasic sites, single strand breaks, DNA protein crosslinking, and oxidation of sugar moieties **(Cooke *et al.*, 2003)**.

- **The impact role of NRF2 in EMT and cancer metastasis**

Nrf2 suppresses immune system against cancer by suppressing myeloid-derived suppressor cells (MDSC) which are a heterogeneous myeloid population containing macrophages, dendritic cells and neutrophils. ROS is an activator of immunosuppression by MDSC which promotes tumor development and metastasis by inhibiting innate and adaptive immunity **(Suzuki *et al.*, 2016)**. These complex interrelated processes require cancer cells to lose contact with their neighboring cells, undergo epithelial-to mesenchymal transition (EMT) and migrate return to their epithelial phenotype (mesenchymal-epithelial transition), and ''seed'' in their new location. Once there, metastatic cells can proliferate to generate secondary tumors. EMT induces changes in the shape and motility of epithelial cells. Once transforming into mesenchymal phenotype, cancer cells lose their cell-cell contact and become mobile and invasive in order to spread into nearby tissues and subsequently distant organs **(Chaffer and Weinberg, 2011)**. Outgrowth at the site of distant dissemination requires metastatic cancer cells to undergo mesenchymal-epithelial transition (MET), a reverse process of EMT, where they regain epithelial properties **(Tsai and Yang, 2013)**. During EMT, epithelial cells lose expression of the adhesion protein E-cadherin in favor of N-cadherin. In cancer cell lines NRF2 promotes EMT by downregulation of E-cadherin expression through unknown mechanisms **(Shen *et al.*, 2014; Arfmann-Knubel *et al.*, 2015)**. Expression of NRF2 is important for the migration of normal and malignant cells, since knockdown of NRF2 greatly impairs migration and invasion of a variety of cell lines **(Zhang *et al.*, 2012; Long *et al.*, 2016)**.

Other studies indicate that NRF2 has anti-metastatic properties. In this context, NRF2 expression in the metastatic microenvironment, and not in the cancer cells, dictates the phenotype. In xenograft models of metastasis, whole-body and myeloid specific NRF2 deletion increases susceptibility to lung metastases due to persistent inflammation and redox alterations in immune cells **(Satoh** *et al.*, **2010; Hiramoto** *et al.*, **2014)**. In contrast, in KEAP1 knockdown mice (Keap1-kd or Keap1f/f), which have reduced expression of KEAP1, or in wild-type mice treated with the NRF2 inducer bardoxolone (CDDO), high NRF2 expression decreases the number of lung metastases **(Hayes and Dinkova-Kostova, 2014; Tebay** *et al.*, **2015; Lee** *et al.*, **2017)**. Disruption of Nrf2 signaling affects the cell cycle progression and proliferation of cancer cell lines in vitro **(Lister** *et al.*, **2011; Ma** *et al.*, **2012)**. Nrf2 silencing in cancer cells causes attenuation of cell migration and tumor metastasis.

- **Regulation of NRF2 by microRNAs**

MicroRNAs (miRNAs) (about 22 – 25 nt) are a class of endogenous small non-coding RNAs that have been found highly conserved among species. MiRNAs are able to negatively regulate gene expression through base pairing of 3' UTRs of their target genes. The miRNAs were known to be involved in distinct steps of metastasis including EMT, migration/invasion, anoikis, survival, intravasation/extravasation and distant organ colonization **(Chan and Wang, 2015).**

The miR-200 family (miR-200a/200b/200c/141/429) has been shown to inhibit cell migration and invasion through targeting ZEB in several cancer types including breast, bladder and ovarian cancers. MiR-200 inhibition was reported to reduce E-cadherin level, thereby increasing cell motility **(Park** *et al.*, **2008)**. On the other hand, it was found that NRF2 was a target for both mir-200a and mir-141, so that mir-200a and mir-141 may affect NRF2 directly or indirectly by targeting Keap1 mRNA **(Duncan** *et al,.* **2015) (Figure 10 and Figure 11)**. Moreover, overexpression of miR-141 activated NF-kB signaling pathway through KEAP1 suppression, while that inhibition of this pathway partially reverses miR-141-mediated cisplatin resistance in ovarian cancer cells **(Van Jaarsveld *et al.*, 2013)**.

MiR-200a/141 is reported to inhibit migration, invasion, proliferation and drug resistance in head and neck squamous cell carcinoma, non-small cell lung cancer, female reproductive cancers and renal cell carcinoma **(Chen *et al.*, 2014)**, but enhance proliferation and drug resistance in colorectal cancer and ovarian cancer **(Hur *et al.*, 2013)**. Further analysis using real time quantitative polymerase chain reaction (RT-qPCR) and luciferase reporter assays revealed that miR-141 exhibited a direct regulatory effect on the downstream Keap1 transcript. Moreover, Shi and colleagues revealed an upregulated expression of miR-141 that correlated with drug resistance to 5-fluorouracil within hepatocellular carcinoma (HCC) cell line chemoresistance models for the drug. In addition, exacerbation of miR-141 function through transient transfection of miR-141mimics allowed for increased chemoresistance to 5-fluorouracil by HCC cell lines **(Shi *et al.*, 2015)**. Totally, mir-141 plays a dual role in tumorigenicity and can modulate cellular motility and control stemness **(Bracken *et al.*, 2008)**.

Overexpression of miR-141 was reported to significantly inhibit the proliferation of gastric cancer (GC). Growth inhibitory effects of miR-141 are in part mediated through its downstream target gene TAZ. TAZ is a transcription cofactor which plays pivotal roles in EMT, cell growth and organ development. TAZ was proposed to endow self-renewal capacity to cancer stem cells and inversely correlated with miR-141 levels in the primary GC tissues **(Cui *et al.*, 2003)**. The *in vitro* angiogenesis role of miR-141 was related to increasing the secretion of VEGFA. What's more, they observed that tumors with high levels of miR-141 had a higher number of blood vessels. It has been revealed that overexpression of miR-141 would lead to overproduction of VEGF-A and increased neoangiogenesis in NSCLC **(Bremnes *et al.*, 2006).**

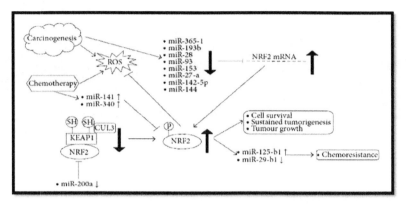

Fig. 10: Overview of carcinogenesis, chemoresistance and the response of NRF2 to dysregulated miRNAs expression.

Besides, Murray-Stewart and colleagues identified miR-200-a as a mediating agent for aiding naturally occurring polyamine analogue-based histone deacetylase inhibitors in reverting chemoresistance properties within non-small-cell lung carcinoma cell lines. The study concluded that the polyamine analogue-induced miR-200-a expression allowed for targeted regulation of Keap1 transcript expression, resulting in NRF2 binding to spermidine/spermine N^1-acetyltransferase (SSAT) promoter regions. Since SSAT is a polyamine catabolic enzyme that plays a major role in chemosensitivity to antitumour drugs, this miRNA/NRF2 interplay leads to lowering the intracellular levels of polyamines within tumour cells and consequently imposing a negative effect on tumour growth **(Murray-Stewart *et al.*, 2013).** Similar evidence for the interplay between miR-200-a and NRF2 was highlighted through the study performed by Eades and colleagues in breast carcinoma cell lines. This study also confirmed that miR-200-a binds successfully to the 3′ UTR of the Keap1 transcript, resulting in direct regulation post-transcriptionally **(Eades *et al.*, 2011).** Another study conducted by Cortez and colleagues recognized the influences of miR-

200c on non-small-cell lung carcinoma cell lines. The results of this study, following miR-200c overexpression, demonstrated the effects of miR-200c on enhancing cell line radiosensitivity through increased apoptotic triggering. In addition, the study also highlighted that miR-200c overexpression had a direct regulatory effect on oxidative stress responses, primarily GABP/NRF2 and SESN1 expression **(Cortez et al., 2014)**. It also was indicated that, the miR-200c and miR-141 cluster (miR-200c/141) could inhibit migration and invasion of gastric cancer by directly targeting of ZEB1 and ZEB2 and the subsequent restoration of E-cadherin **(Bullock et al., 2012)**.

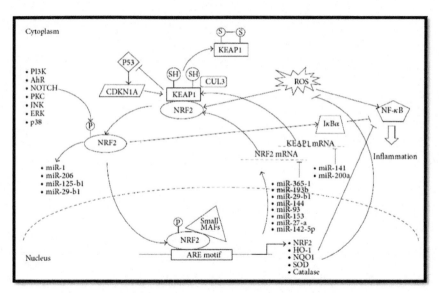

Fig.11: Regulatory mechanisms of NRF2, highlighting miRNA-mediated influences. Important regulatory pathways include the inhibition of NF-*k*B proinflammatory and ROS pathways.

Mir-34a that was improved to indirect regulate NRF2 via repression of Sirt1 (repressor of NRF2), Siemens and colleagues showed that ectopic expression of miR-34a, a P53-regulated microRNA, leading to inhibition of EMT phenotypes including migration and invasion, by down regulation of Snail levels **(Siemens et al., 2011)**.

While miR-21, the first "oncomiR" to be identified and regulated by NF-*k*B, was shown to play a role in promoting EMT. Inhibition of miR-21 using antagomir in MDA-MB-231 invasive breast cancer cells was able to reverse EMT and cancer stem cell (CSC) phenotype by up-regulation of PTEN, leading to inactivation of AKT/ERK **(Han et al., 2012)**. It also has been shown to serve as an indicator of poor prognosis in various cancer types, including breast **(Qian et al., 2009)**, liver **(Jiang et al., 2008)**, lung **(Markou et al., 2008)**, and colorectal cancer **(Schetter et al., 2008)**.

Previous studies have shown that miR-146 induction depends on NF-κB activation **(Taganov et al., 2006)**. A subsequent investigation demonstrated that miR-146a/b suppressed breast cancer metastasis via reducing the activity of NF-κB by directly targeting IRAK1 and TRAF6, both of which are known to positively regulate NF-κB activity **(Bhaumik et al., 2008)**. Those findings suggest that NF-κB and miR-146 form a negative regulatory loop.

A recent study demonstrated that, mir-500a-5p overexpression in ER+ breast cancer cell lines resulted in downregulation of transcripts (SLC7A11, TXNRD1 "Thioredoxin Reductase 1", GPX2, PTGR1, HMOX1, ABCC2, and UGT1A6) belonging to oxidative stress/NRF2 pathways and specifically known targets of NRF2 **(Esposti et al., 2017)**. Also, currently, only three genes which are negative regulators of NF-kB signaling (namely *CYLD*, *TAX1BP1* and *OTUD7B*) have been discovered as validated targets for miR-500a in gastric cancer **(Zhang et al., 2015)**.

- # References

Arai T., Miyoshi Y. and Kim S.J. (2008): Association of GSTP1 expression with resistance to docetaxel and paclitaxel in human breast cancers. *Eur J Surg Oncol*; 34:734–738.

Arfmann-Knubel S., Struck B., Genrich G., Helm O., Sipos B., Sebens S., and Schafer H. (2015): The crosstalk between Nrf2 and TGF-beta1 in the epithelial-mesenchymal transition of pancreatic duct epithelial cells. *PLoS One*; 10, e0132978.

Arguello F., Baggs R.B., Eskenazi A.E., Duerst R.E. and Frantz C.N. (1991): Vascular anatomy and organspecific tumor growth as critical factors in the development of metastases and their distribution among organs. *Int J Cancer*; 48:583–90.

Asher G., Lotem J., Cohen B., Sachs L. and Shaul Y. (2001): Regulation of p53 stability and p53-dependent apoptosis by NADH quinone oxidoreductase 1. *Proc Natl Acad Sci U S A*; 98(3):1188-1193.

Asher G., Lotem J., Sachs L., Kahana C. and Shaul Y. (2002): Mdm- 2 and ubiquitin-independent p53 proteasomal degradation regulated by NQO1. *Proc Natl Acad Sci U S A*; 99(20):13125-13130.

Asher G., Tsvetkov P., Kahana C. and Shaul Y. (2005): A mechanism of ubiquitin-independent proteasomal degradation of the tumor suppressors p53 and p73. *Genes Dev*; 19(3):316-321.

Bailey-Downs L.C., Mitschelen M., Sosnowska D., Toth P., Pinto J.T., Ballabh P., Valcarcel-Ares M.N., Farley J., Koller A., Henthorn J.C., Bass C., Sonntag W.E., Ungvari Z. and Csiszar A. (2012): Liver-specific knockdown of IGF-1 decreases vascular oxidative stress resistance by impairing the Nrf2-dependent antioxidant response: a novel model of vascular aging. *J Gerontol A Biol Sci Med Sci*; 67:313–329.

Ballatori N., Hammond C.L.and Cunningham J.B. (2005): Molecular mechanisms of reduced glutathione transport: role of the MRP/CFTR/ABCC and OATP/SLC21A families of membrane proteins. *Toxicol Appl Pharmacol*; 204:238–255.

Benson A.M., Hunkeler M.J. and Talalay P. (1980): Increase of NAD(P)H:quinone reductase by dietary antioxidants: possible role in protection against carcinogenesis and toxicity. *Proc Natl Acad Sci USA*; 77:5216–5220.

Bhaumik D., Scott G.K., Schokrpur S., Patil C.K., Campisi J. and Benz C.C. (2008): Expression of microRNA-146 suppresses NF-kappaB activity with reduction of metastatic potential in breast cancer cells. *Oncogene*; 27:5643–7.

Bonello S., Zähringer C., BelAiba R.S., Djordjevic T., Hess J., Michiels C., Kietzmann T., and Görlach A. (2007): Reactive Oxygen Species Activate the HIF-1α Promoter Via a Functional NF-kB Site. *Arterioscler. Thromb. Vasc. Biol.*; 27, 755–761.

Bracken C.P., Gregory P.A., Kolesnikoff N., Bert A.G., Wang J., Shannon M.F. and Goodall G.J. (2008): A double-negative feedback loop between ZEB1-SIP1 and the microRNA-200 family regulates epithelial-mesenchymal transition. *Cancer Res*; 68:7846-7854.

Breimer L.H. (1990): Molecular mechanisms of oxygen radical carcinogenesis andmutagenesis: the role of DNA base damage. *Mol. Carcinog*; 3 (4), 188–197.

Bremnes R.M., Camps C. and Sirera R (2006): Angiogenesis in non-small cell lung cancer: the prognostic impact of neoangiogenesis and the cytokines VEGF and bFGF in tumours and blood. *Lung Cancer*; 51:143-158.

Bryan H.K., Olayanju A., Goldring C.E. and Park B.K. (2013): The Nrf2 cell defence pathway: Keap1-dependent and -independent mechanisms of regulation. *Biochem. Pharmacol.*; 85, 705–717.

Bullock M.D., Sayan A.E., Packham G.K. and Mirnezami A.H. (2012): MicroRNAs: critical regulators of epithelial to mesenchymal (EMT) and mesenchymal to epithelial transition (MET) in cancer progression. *Biol Cell*; 104:3-12.

Chaffer C.L. and Weinberg R.A. (2011): A perspective on cancer cell metastasis. *Science*; 331:1559–64.

Chan S. and Wang L. (2015): Regulation of cancer metastasis by microRNAs. *Journal of Biomedical Science*; 22:9.

Chen N., Yi X., Abushahin N., Pang S., Zhang D., Kong B. and Zheng W. (2011): Nrf2 expression in endometrial serous carcinomas and its precancers. *Int J Clin Exp Pathol.*; 4:85–96.

Chen W., Sun Z., Wang X.J., Jiang T., Huang Z., Fang D. and Zhang D.D. (2009): Direct interaction between Nrf2 and p21 (Cip1/ WAF1) upregulates the Nrf2-mediated antioxidant response. *Mol Cell*; 34(6):663-673.

Chen X., Wang X., Ruan A., Han W., Zhao Y., Lu X., Xiao P., Shi H., Wang R., Chen L., Chen S., Du Q., Yang H. and Zhang X. (2014): miR-141 is a key regulator of renal cell carcinoma proliferation and metastasis by controlling EphA2 expression. *Clin Cancer Res*; 20:2617-2630.

Chen X.L. and Kunsch C. (2004): Induction of cytoprotective genes through Nrf2/antioxidant response element pathway: a new therapeutic approach for the treatment of inflammatory diseases. *Curr Pharm Des*; 10:879–891.

Chen Z.S., Furukawa T. and Sumizawa T. (1999): ATP-dependent efflux of CPT-11 and SN-38 by the multidrug resistance protein (MRP) and its inhibition by PAK-104P. *Mol Pharmacol*; 55:921–928.

Choi K., Ryu S.W., Song S., Choi H., Kang S.W. and Choi C. (2010): Caspase-dependent generation of reactive oxygen species in human astrocytoma cells contributes to resistance to TRAIL-mediated apoptosis. *Cell Death Differ*; 17(5):833-845.

Choi B.-h. and Kwak M.-K. (2016): Shadows of NRF2 in cancer: resistance to chemotherapy. *Curr. Opin. Toxicol.* 1, 20-28.

Cipolla C.M. and Lodhi I.J. (2017): Peroxisomal dysfunction in age-related diseases. *Trends Endocrinol. Metab*; 28, 297–308.

Cooke M.S., Evans M.D., Dizdaroglu M. and Lunec J. (2003): Oxidative DNA damage: mechanisms, mutation, and disease. *FASEB J*; 17, 1195–1214.

Cortez M., Valdecanas D. and Zhang X. (2014): Therapeutic delivery of miR-200c enhances radiosensitity in lung cancer. MolecularTherapy; 22 (8): 1494–1503.

Cui C.B., Cooper L.F., Yang X., Karsenty G. and Aukhil I (2003): Transcriptional coactivation of bone-specific transcription factor Cbfa1 by TAZ. *Mol Cell Biol*; 23:1004-1013.

Danza K., Silvestris N., Simone G., Signorile M., Saragoni L., Brunetti O., Monti M., Mazzotta A., De Summa S and Mangia A. (2016): Role of miR-27a, miR-181a and miR-20b in gastric cancer hypoxia-induced chemoresistance. *Cancer Biol. Ther*; 17, 400–406.

Das U., Manna K., Khan A., Sinha M., Biswas S., Sengupta A., Chakraborty A. and Dey S. (2017): Ferulic acid (FA) abrogates gamma-radiation induced oxidative stress and DNA damage by up-regulating nuclear translocation of Nrf2 and activation of NHEJ pathway. *Free Radic. Res*; 51, 47–63.

Degradation H., De Luca P., Zalazar F., Coluccio-leskow F., Meiss R., Navone N., De Siervi A., Elguero B, Gueron G. and Giudice, J. (2012): De Unveiling the association of STAT3 and HO-1 in prostate cancer: role beyond heme degradation. *Neoplasia*; 14, 1043–1056.

Ding Z., Yang L., Xie X., Xie F., Pan F., Li J., He J. and Liang H. (2003): Expression and significance of resistance protein BCRP (ABCG2). *Oncogene*; 22:7340–7358.

Du Z.X., Yan Y., Zhang H.Y., Liu B.Q., Gao Y.Y., Niu X.F., Meng X. and Wang H.Q. (2011): Proteasome inhibition induces a p38 MAPK pathway-dependent antiapoptotic program via Nrf2 in thyroid cancer cells. *J Clin Endocrinol Metab*; 96:E763–E771.

Duckers H.J., Boehm M., True A.L., Yet S.F., San H., Park J.L., Clinton Webb R., Lee M.E., Nabel G.J. and Nabel E.G. (2001): Heme oxygenase-1 protects against vascular constriction and proliferation. *Nat Med*; 7:693–698.

Dulak J., Deshane J., Jozkowicz A. and Agarwal A. (2008): Heme oxygenase-1 and carbon monoxide in vascular pathobiology: focus on angiogenesis. *Circulation*; 117:231–241.

Dulak J., Jozkowicz A., Foresti R., Kasza A., Frick M., Huk I., Green C.J., Pachinger O., Weidinger F. and Motterlini R. (2002): Heme oxygenase activity modulates vascular endothelial growth factor synthesis in vascular smooth muscle cells. *Antioxid Redox Signal*; 4:229–240.

Duncan A., Byron B. and Therese H. (2015): miRNA Influences in NRF2 Pathway Interactions within Cancer Models. *Journal of Nucleic Acids*; http://dx.doi.org/10.1155/2015/143636

Duong H.Q., Yi Y.W. and Kang H.J. (2014): Inhibition of NRF2 by PIK-75 augments sensitivity of pancreatic cancer cells to gemcitabine. *Int J Oncol*; 44:959–969.

Eades G., Yang M., Yao Y., Zhang Y., and Zhou Q. (2011): miR-200a regulates Nrf2 activation by targeting Keap1 mRNA in breast cancer cells. *Journal of Biological Chemistry*; 286 (47): 40725–40733.

El-Deiry W.S., Tokino T., Velculescu V.E., Levy D.B., Parsons R., Trent J.M., Lin D., Mercer W.E., Kinzler K.W. and Vogelstein B. (1993): WAF1, a potential mediator of p53 tumor suppression. *Cell*; 75(4):817-825.

Esposti D., Aushev V. N., Lee E., Cros M., Zhu J., Herceg Z., Chen J. and Hernandez-Vargas H. (2017): miR-500a-5p regulates oxidative stress response genes in breast cancer and predicts cancer survival. *Scientific Reports*; 7: 15966.

Ferrara N., Gerber H.P. and LeCouter J. (2003): The biology of VEGF and its receptors. *Nat Med*; 9:669–676.

Folkman J. and Shing Y. (1992): Angiogenesis. *J Biol Chem*; 267:10931–10934.

Görlach A. (2014): Hypoxia and Reactive Oxygen Species. In Hypoxia and Cancer; Melillo G., Ed.; *Springer: New York, NY, USA*; pp. 65–90.

Gorrini C., Harris I.S. and Mak T.W. (2013): Modulation of oxidative stress as an anticancer strategy. *Nat. Rev. Drug Discov*; 12, 931–947.

Guan S. Tee, W., Ng D., Chan T., Peh H., Ho W., Cheng C., Mak J., Wong W. and Fred Wong W. (2013): Andrographolide protects against cigarette smoke-induced oxidative lung injury via augmentation of Nrf2 activity. *Br. J. Pharmacol*; 168, 1707–1718.

Han M., Liu M., Wang Y., Chen X., Xu J. and Sun Y. (2012): Antagonism of miR-21 reverses epithelial-mesenchymal transition and cancer stem cell phenotype through AKT/ERK1/2 inactivation by targeting PTEN. *PLoS One*; 7:e39520.

Hayes J.D. and Dinkova-Kostova A.T. (2014): The Nrf2 regulatory network provides an interface between redox and intermediary metabolism. *Trends Biochem Sci*; 39:199–218.

Hayes J.D., Flanagan J.U. and Jowsey I.R. (2005): Glutathione transferases. *Annu Rev Pharmacol Toxicol*; 45:51–88.

He X., Wang J., Wei W., Shi M., Xin B., Zhan, T. and Shen X. (2016): Hypoxia regulates ABCG2 activity through the activation of ERK1/2/HIF-1_ and contributes to chemoresistance in pancreatic cancer cells. *Cancer Biol. Ther*; 17, 188–198.

Heasman S.A., Zaitseva L. and Bowles K.M. (2011): Protection of acute myeloid leukaemia cells from apoptosis induced by front-line chemotherapeutics is mediated by haem oxygenase-1. *Oncotarget*; 2:658–668.

Hicklin D.J. and Ellis L.M. (2005): Role of the vascular endothelial growth factor pathway in tumor growth and angiogenesis. *J Clin Oncol*; 23:1011–1027.

Hillen F. and Griffioen A.W. (2007): Tumour vascularization: sprouting angiogenesis and beyond. *Cancer Metastasis Rev*; 26:489–502.

Hiramoto K., Satoh H., Suzuki T., Moriguchi T., Pi J., Shimosegawa T., and Yamamoto M. (2014): Myeloid lineage-specific deletion of antioxidant system enhances tumor metastasis. *Cancer Prev. Res. (Phila.)*; 7, 835–844.

Hooijberg J.H., Broxterman H.J. and Kool M. (1999): Antifolate resistance mediated by the multidrug resistance proteins MRP1 and MRP2. *Cancer Res*; 59:2532–2535.

Huang J., Tan P.H. and Thiyagarajan J. (2003): Prognostic significance of glutathione S-transferase-pi in invasive breast cancer. *Mod Pathol*; 16:558–565.

Huang Y. and Sadee W. (2006): Membrane transporters and channels in chemoresistance and -sensitivity of tumor cells. *Cancer Lett*; 239:168–182.

Hur K., Toiyama Y., Takahashi M., Balaguer F., Nagasaka T., Koike J., Hemmi H., Koi M., Boland C.R. and Goel A. (2013): MicroRNA-200c modulates epithelial-to-mesenchymal transition (EMT) in human colorectal cancer metastasis. *Gut*; 62:1315-1326.

Hwang A.B. and Lee S.J. (2011): Regulation of life span by mitochondrial respiration: the HIF-1 and ROS connection. *Aging (Albany NY)*; 3(3):304-310.

Ikeda H., Nishi S. and Sakai M. (2004): Transcription factor Nrf2/MafK regulates ratplacental glutathione S-transferase gene during hepato-carcinogenesis. *Biochem. J*; 380 (2), 515–521.

Jaiswal A.K. (2004): Nrf2 signaling in coordinated activation of antioxidant geneexpression. Free Radic. *Biol. Med*; 36 (10), 1199–1207.

Jayakumar S., Pal D., and Sandur S.K. (2015): Nrf2 facilitates repair of radiation induced DNA damage through homologous recombination repair pathway in a ROS independent manner in cancer cells. *Mutat. Res*; 779, 33–45.

Jazwa A., Loboda A., Golda S., Cisowski J., Szelag M., Zagorska A., Sroczynska P., Drukala J., Jozkowicz A. and Dulak J. (2006): Effect of heme and heme oxygenase-1 on vascular endothelial growth factor synthesis and angiogenic potency of human keratinocytes. *Free Radic Biol Med*; 40:1250–1263.

Jeon W.K., Hong H.Y. and Seo W.C. (2012): Smad7 sensitizes A549 lung cancer cells to cisplatin-induced apoptosis through heme oxygenase-1 inhibition. *Biochem Biophys Res Commun*; 420:288–292.

Ji X. *et al.* (2014): Knockdown of Nrf2 suppresses glioblastoma angiogenesis by inhibiting hypoxia-induced activation of HIF-1alpha. *Int J Cancer*; 135: 574–584.

Ji, X. J. *et al.*(2013): Knockdown of NF-E2-related factor 2 inhibits the proliferation and growth of U251MG human glioma cells in a mouse xenograft model. *Oncol Rep*; 30: 157–164.

Jia Y., Wang H., Wang Q., Ding H., Wu H. and Pan H. (2016): Silencing Nrf2 impairs glioma cell proliferation via AMPK-activated mTOR inhibition. *Biochem. Biophys. Res. Commun*; 469: 665-671.

Jiang J., Gusev Y., Aderca I., Mettler T.A., Nagorney D.M. and Brackett D.J. (2008): Association of MicroRNA expression in hepatocellular carcinomas with hepatitis infection, cirrhosis, and patient survival. *Clin Cancer Res*; 14:419–27.

Jiang L., Shestov A.A., Swain P., Yang C., Parker S.J., Wang Q.A., Terada L.S., Adams N.D., McCabe M.T. and Pietrak B. (2016): Reductive carboxylation supports redox homeostasis during anchorage-independent growth. *Nature*; 532: 255–258.

Johansson K., Ahlen K. and Rinaldi R. (2007): Microsomal glutathione transferase 1 in anticancer drug resistance. *Carcinogenesis*; 28:465–470.

Johansson K., Jarvliden J. and Gogvadze V. (2010): Multiple roles of microsomal glutathione transferase 1 in cellular protection: a mechanistic study. *Free Radic Biol Med*; 49:1638–1645.

Jozkowicz A., Huk I., Nigisch A., Weigel G., Dietrich W., Motterlini R. and Dulak J. (2003): Heme oxygenase and angiogenic activity of endothelial cells: stimulation by carbon monoxide and inhibition by tin protoporphyrin-IX. *Antioxid Redox Signal*; 5:155–162.

Jozkowicz A., Was H. and Dulak J. (2007): Heme oxygenase-1 in tumors: is it a falsefriend? Antioxid. Redox. *Signal*; 9 (12): 2099–2118.

Kalo E., Kogan-Sakin I., Solomon H., Bar-Nathan E., Shay M., Shetzer Y., Dekel E., Goldfinger N., Buganim Y., Stambolsky P., Goldstein I., Madar S. and Rotter V. (2012): Mutant p53R273H attenuates the expression of phase 2 detoxifying enzymes and promotes the survival of cells with high ROS levels. *J Cell Sci.*

Kim T. H. *et al.* (2011): NRF2 blockade suppresses colon tumor angiogenesis by inhibiting hypoxia-induced activation of HIF-1alpha. *Anticancer Res*; 71, 2260–2275.

Konstantinopoulos P.A., Spentzos D., Fountzilas E., Francoeur N., Sanisetty S., Grammatikos A.P., Hecht J.L. and Cannistra S.A. (2011): Keap1 mutations and Nrf2 pathway activation in epithelial ovarian cancer. *Cancer Res*; 71: 5081– 5089.

Krock B.L., Skuli N. and Simon M.C. (2011): Hypoxia-induced angiogenesis: Good and evil. *Genes Cancer*; 2: 1117–1133.

Lavrovsky Y., Schwartzmant M.L., Levere R.D., Kappas A. and Abraham N.G. (1994): Identification of binding sites for transcription factors NF-kappa B and AP-2 in the promoter region of the human heme oxygenase 1 gene (eyhroeukemlc c/stre proein/derenatn). *Cell Biol*; 91: 5987–5991.

Lee J.S. and Surh Y.J. (2005): Nrf2 as a novel molecular target for chemoprevention. *Cancer Lett*; 224:171–184.

Lee S.B., Kim C.Y., Lee H.J., Yun J.H. and Nho C.W. (2009): Induction of the phase IIdetoxification enzyme NQO1 in hepatocarcinoma cells by lignans from thefruit of Schisandra chinensis through nuclear accumulation of Nrf2. *PlantaMed*; 75 (12): 1314–1318.

Lee S.B., Sellers B.N., and Denicola G.M. (2017): The regulation of NRF2 by nutrient-responsive signaling and its role in anabolic cancer metabolism. *Antioxid. Redox Signal.*

Lewis D.F. (2004): 57 varieties: the human cytochromes P450. *Pharmacogenomics*; 5:305–318.

Li Volti G., Sacerdoti D., Sangras B., Vanella A., Mezentsev A., Scapagnini G., Falck J.R. and Abraham N.G. (2005): Carbon monoxide signaling in promoting angiogenesis in human microvessel endothelial cells. *Antioxid Redox Signal*; 7:704–710.

Li L., Pan H., Wang H., Li X., Bu X., Wang Q., Gao Y., Wen G., Zhou Y., Cong Z. (2016): Interplay between VEGF and Nrf2 regulates angiogenesis due to intracranial venous hypertension. *Sci. Rep*; 6: 37338.

Li Y., Su J., DingZhang X., Zhang J., Yoshimoto M., Liu S., Bijian K., Gupta A., Squire J.A., Alaoui Jamali M.A. and Bismar T.A. (2011): PTEN deletion and heme oxygenase-1 overexpression cooperate in prostate cancer progression and are associated with adverse clinical outcome. *J. Pathol*; 224: 90–100.

Lili J., Wei Y. and Jiang T. (2014): Correlation of Nrf2, NQO1, MRP1, cmyc and p53 in colorectal cancer and their relationships to clinicopathologic features and survival. *Int J Clin Exp Pathol*; 7:1124–1131.

Lin H.-C., Su S.-L., Lu C.-Y., Lin A.-H., Lin W.-C., Liu C.-S., Yang Y.-C., Wang H.-M., Lii C.-K. and Chen H.-W. (2017): Andrographolide inhibits hypoxia-induced HIF-1_-driven endothelin 1 secretion by activating Nrf2/HO-1 and promoting the expression of prolyl hydroxylases 2/3 in human endothelial cells. *Environ. Toxicol*; 32: 918–930.

Liu L., Ning X., Sun L., Zhang H., Shi Y., Guo C., Han S., Liu J., Sun S. and Han Z. (2008): Hypoxia-inducible factor-1 alpha contributes to hypoxia-induced chemoresistance in gastric cancer. *Cancer Sci*; 99: 121–128.

Lister A., Nedjadi T., Kitteringham N.R., Campbell F., Costello E., Lloyd B., Copple I.M., Williams S., Owen A. and Neoptolemos J.P. (2011): Nrf2 is overexpressed in pancreatic cancer: implications for cell proliferation and therapy. *Mol. Cancer*; 10-37.

Liwen L., Pan H., Wang H., Li X., Bu X., Wang Q., Gao Y., Wen G., Zhou Y., Cong Z., Yang Y., Tang C. and Liu Z. (2016): Interplay between VEGF anf Nrf2 regulates angiogenesis due to intracranial venous hypertension. *Science REPORTS*; 6: 37338.

Loboda A., Stachurska A., Florczyk U., Rudnicka D., Jazwa A.,Wegrzyn J., Kozakowska M., Stalinska K., Poellinger L. and Levonen A. (2009): HIF-1 induction attenuates Nrf2-dependent IL-8 expression in human endothelial cells. *Antioxid. Redox Signal*; 11: 1501–1517.

Long D.J., Waikel R.L., Wang X.J., Perlaky L., Roop D.R. and Jaiswal A.K. (2000): NAD(P)H:quinone oxidoreductase 1 deficiency increases susceptibility to benzo(a)pyrene-induced mouse skin carcinogenesis. *Cancer Res*; 60:5913–5915.

Long M., Rojo de la Vega M., Wen Q., Bharara M., Jiang T., Zhang R., Zhou S., Wong P.K., Wondrak G.T., Zheng H., and Zhang, D.D. (2016): An essential role of NRF2 in diabetic wound healing. *Diabetes*; 65: 780–793.

Ma R., Zhang M., Wang J., Cai H., Yeer M. and Duan X. (2010): [Expression and distribution of Nrf2 in several hepatocellular carcinoma cell lines]. hypoxia-inducible factor-1 alpha and MDR1/P-glycoprotein in human colon carcinoma tissue and cells. *J. Cancer Res. Clin. Oncol*; 136: 1697–1707.

Ma X., Zhang J., Liu S., Huang Y., Chen B., and Wang D. (2012): Nrf2 knockdown by shRNA inhibits tumor growth and increases efficacy of chemotherapy in cervical cancer. *Cancer Chemother. Pharmacol*; 69: 485–494.

Ma Y. and Wink M. (2010): The beta-carboline alkaloid harmine inhibits BCRP and can reverse resistance to the anticancer drugs mitoxantrone and camptothecin in breast cancer cells. *Phytother Res*; 24:146–149.

Mahaffey C.M., Mahaffey N.C. and Holland W. (2012): Aberrant regulation of the MRP3 gene in non-small cell lung carcinoma. *J Thorac Oncol*; 7:34–39.

Mahaffey C.M., Zhang H. and Rinna A. (2009): Multidrug-resistant protein-3 gene regulation by the transcription factor Nrf2 in human bronchial epithelial and non-small-cell lung carcinoma. *Free Radic Biol Med*; 46:1650–1657.

Mahaffey C.M., Zhang H., Rinna A., Holland W., Mack P.C. and Forman H.J. (2009): Multidrug-resistant protein-3 gene regulation by the transcription factor Nrf2in human bronchial epithelial and non-small-cell lung carcinoma. *Free Radic.Biol. Med*; 46 (12): 1650–1657.

Maliepaard M., van Gastelen M.A. and Tohgo A. (2001): Circumvention of breast cancer resistance protein (BCRP)- mediated resistance to camptothecins in vitro using nonsubstrate drugs or the BCRP inhibitor GF1209181. *Clin Cancer Res*; 7:935–941.

Malinin N.L., West X.Z. and Byzova T.V. (2011): Oxidation as "the stress of life". *Aging (Albany NY)*; 3(9):906-910.

Markou A., Tsaroucha E.G., Kaklamanis L., Fotinou M., Georgoulias V. and Lianidou E.S. (2008): Prognostic value of mature microRNA-21 and microRNA-205 overexpression in non-small cell lung cancer by quantitative real-time RT-PCR. *Clin Chem*; 54:1696–704.

Mayerhofer M., Florian S. and Krauth M.T. (2004): Identification of heme oxygenase-1 as a novel BCR/ABLdependent survival factor in chronic myeloid leukemia. *Cancer Res*; 64:3148–3154.

Meijerman I., Beijnen J.H. and Schellens J.H. (2008): Combined action and regulation ofphase II enzymes and multidrug resistance proteins in multidrug resistance incancer. *Cancer Treat Rev*; 34 (6): 505–520.

Meng D., Wang X., Chang Q., Hitron A., Zhang Z., Xu M., Chen G., Luo J., Jiang B., Fang J. and Shi X. (2010): Arsenic promotes angiogenesis *in vitro* via a heme oxygenase-1-dependent mechanism. *Toxicol Appl Pharmacol*; 244:291–299.

Miyake M., Fujimoto K., Anai S., Ohnishi S., Kuwada M., Nakai Y., Inoue T., Matsumura Y., Tomioka A. and Ikeda T. (2011): Heme oxygenase-1 promotes angiogenesis in urothelial carcinoma of the urinary bladder. *Oncol. Rep*; 25: 653–660.

Motohashi H., O'Connor T., Katsuoka F., Engel J.D. and Yamamoto M. (2002): Integration and diversity of the regulatory network composed of Maf and CNC families of transcription factors. *Gene*; 294:1–12.

Murray-Stewart T., Hanigan C., Woster P., Marton L., and Casero R. (2013): Histone deacetylase inhibition overcomes drug resistance through a miRNA-dependent mechanism. *Molecular Cancer Therapeutics*; 12 (10): 2088–2099.

Muz B., de la Puente P., Azab F., and Azab A.K. (2015): The role of hypoxia in cancer progression, angiogenesis, metastasis, and resistance to therapy. *Hypoxia (Auckl.)*; 3: 83–92.

Nebert D.W., Wikvall K. and Miller W.L. (2013): Human cytochromes P450 in health and disease. *Philos Trans R Soc Lond B Biol Sci*; 368:20120431.

Nemeth Z., Li M., Csizmadia E., Dome B., Johansson M., Persson J.L., Seth P., Otterbein L. and Wegiel B. (2015): Heme oxygenase-1 in macrophages controls prostate cancer progression. *Oncotarget*; 6: 33675–33688.

Nishikawa S., Konno M., Hamabe A., et al. (2013): Aldehyde dehydrogenase high gastric cancer stem cells are resistant to chemotherapy. *Int J Oncol*; 42:1437–1442.

Noda E., Maeda K., Inoue T., et al. (2012): Predictive value of expression of ERCC 1 and GST-p for 5-fluorouracil/oxaliplatin chemotherapy in advanced colorectal cancer. *Hepatogastroenterology*; 59:130–133.

North S., Moenner M. and Bikfalvi A. (2005): Recent developments in the regulation of the angiogenic switch by cellular stress factors in tumors. *Cancer Lett*; 218:1–14.

Nowis D., Bugajski M., Winiarska M., et al. (2008): Zinc protoporphyrin IX, a heme oxygenase-1 inhibitor, demonstrates potent antitumor effects but is unable to potentiate antitumor effects of chemotherapeutics in mice. *BMC Cancer*; 8:197.

Oguri T., Isobe T., Suzuki T., et al. (2000): Increased expression of the MRP5 gene is associated with exposure to platinum drugs in lung cancer. *Int J Cancer*; 86:95–100.

Oh E.T., Kim J.W., Kim J.M., Kim S.J., Lee J.S., Hong S.S., Goodwin J., Ruthenborg R.J., Jung M.G. and Lee H.J. (2016): NQO1 inhibits proteasome-mediated degradation of HIF-1alpha. *Nat. Commun*; 7: 13593.

Palazon A., Goldrath A.W., Nizet V. and Johnson R.S. (2014): HIF Transcription Factors, Inflammation, and Immunity. *Immunity*; 41: 518–528.

Pang L.Y., Scott M., Hayward R.L., Mohammed H., Whitelaw C.B., Smith G.C. and Hupp T.R. (2011): p21 (WAF1) is component of a positive feedback loop that maintains the p53 transcriptional program. *Cell Cycle*; 10(6):932-950.

Park S.M., Gaur A.B., Lengyel E. and Peter M.E. (2008): The miR-200 family determines the epithelial phenotype of cancer cells by targeting the E-cadherin repressors ZEB1 and ZEB2. *Genes Dev*; 22:894–907.

Pölönen P. and Levonen A.L. (2016): Insights into the role of NRF2 in cancer provided by cancer genomics. *Curr. Opin. Toxicol*; 1: 111–117.

Qian B., Katsaros D., Lu L., Preti M., Durando A., Arisio R., et al. (2009): High miR-21 expression in breast cancer associated with poor disease-free survival in early stage disease and high TGF-beta1. *Breast Cancer Res Treat*; 117:131–40.

Rankin E.B. and Giaccia A.J. (2016): Hypoxic control of metastasis. *Science*; 352: 175–180.

Robey R.W., Medina-P_erez W.Y., Nishiyama K., et al. (2001): Overexpression of the ATP-binding cassette half-transporter, ABCG2 (MXR/BCRP/ABCP1), in flavopiridol-resistant human breast cancer cells. *Clin Cancer Res*; 7:145–152.

Rotblat B., Melino G. and Knight R. (2012): NRF2 and P53: Januses in cancer?. *Oncotarget*; 3:1272-1283.

Sasaki H., Shitara M., Yokota K., et al. (2012): MRP3 gene expression correlates with NRF2 mutations in lung squamous cell carcinomas. *Mol Med Rep*; 6:705–708.

Satoh,H., Moriguchi T., Takai J., Ebina M., and Yamamoto M. (2013): Nrf2 prevents initiation but accelerates progression through the Kras signaling pathway during lung carcinogenesis. *Cancer Res*; 73: 4158–4168.

Saxena M., Stephens M.A., Pathak H. and Rangarajan A. (2011): Transcription factors that mediate epithelial-mesenchymal transition lead to multidrug resistance by upregulating ABC transporters. *Cell Death Dis*; 2:e179.

Schafer A., Teufel J., Ringel F., et al. (2012): Aldehyde dehydrogenase 1A1-a new mediator of resistance to temozolomide in glioblastoma. *Neuro-oncology*; 14:1452–1464.

Schetter A.J., Leung S.Y., Sohn J.J., Zanetti K.A., Bowman E.D., Yanaihara N., et al. (2008): MicroRNA expression profiles associated with prognosis and therapeutic outcome in colon adenocarcinoma. *JAMA*; 299:425–36.

Scotlandi K., Remondini D., Castellani G., et al. (2009): Overcoming resistance to conventional drugs in Ewing sarcoma and identification of molecular predictors of outcome. *J Clin Oncol*; 27:2209–2216.

Shi L., Wu L. and Chen Z. (2015): MiR-141 activates Nrf2-dependent antioxidant pathway via down-regulating the expression of keap1 conferring the resistance of hepatocellular carcinoma cells to 5-fluorouracil. *Cellular Physiology and Biochemistry*; 35 (6): 2333–2348.

Shim G.S., Manandhar S., Shin D.H., et al. (2009): Acquisition of doxorubicin resistance in ovarian carcinoma cells accompanies activation of the NRF2 pathway. *Free Radic Biol Med*; 47:1619–1631.

Siemens H., Jackstadt R., Hunten S., Kaller M., Menssen A., Gotz U., et al. (2011): miR-34 and SNAIL form a double-negative feedback loop to regulate epithelialmesenchymal transitions. *Cell Cycle*; 10:4256–71.

Singh A., Wu H., Zhang P., et al. (2010): Expression of ABCG2 (BCRP) is regulated by Nrf2 in cancer cells that confers side population and chemoresistance phenotype. *Mol Cancer Ther*; 9:2365–2376.

Singh A., Misra V., Thimmulappa R.K., Lee H., Ames S., Hoque M.O., Herman J.G., Baylin S.B., Sidransky D., Gabrielson, E. et al. (2006): Dysfunctional KEAP1-NRF2 interaction in non-small-cell lung cancer. *PLoS Med*; 3: e420.

Solis L.M., Behrens C., Dong W., Suraokar M., Ozburn N.C., Moran C.A., Corvalan A.H., Biswal S., Swisher S.G. and Bekele B.N. (2010): Nrf2 and Keap1 Abnormalities in Non–Small Cell Lung Carcinoma and Association with Clinicopathologic Features. *Clin Cancer Res*; 16:3743–3753.

Sporn M.B. and Liby K.T. (2012): NRF2 and cancer: the good, the bad and the importance of context. *Nature Reviews Cancer*; 12: 564–571.

Su F., Hu X., Jia W., et al. (2003): Glutathion s transferase pi indicates chemotherapy resistance in breast cancer. *J Surg Res*; 113:102–108.

Sun Y., Guan Z., Liang L., Cheng Y., Zhou J., Li J. and Xu, Y. (2016): HIF-1α/MDR1 pathway confers chemoresistance to cisplatin in bladder cancer. *Oncol. Rep*; 35: 1549–1556.

Suzuki M., Otsuki A., Keleku-Lukwete N. and Yamamoto M. (2016): Overview of redox regulation by Keap1–Nrf2 system in toxicology. *Curr. Opin. Toxicol* and cancer; 1: 29–36.

Syu J.-P., Chi J.-T., Kung H.-N., Syu J.-P., Chi J.-T. and Kung H.-N. (2016): Nrf2 is the key to chemotherapy resistance in MCF7 breast cancer cells under hypoxia. *Oncotarget*; 7: 14659–14672.

Taganov K.D., Boldin M.P., Chang K.J. and Baltimore D. (2006): NF-kappaB-dependent induction of microRNA miR-146, an inhibitor targeted to signaling proteins of innate immune responses. *Proc Natl Acad Sci U S A*; 103:12481–6.

Tao S., Rojo de la Vega M., Chapman E., Ooi A., and Zhang D.D. (2017): The effects of NRF2 modulation on the initiation and progression of chemically and genetically induced lung cancer. *Mol. Carcinog*; 57: 182–192.

Toth R.K. and Warfel N.A. (2017): Stange Bedfellows: Nuclear Factor, Erythroid 2-Like 2 (Nrf2) and Hypoxia-Inducible Factor 1 (HIF-1) in Tumor Hypoxia. *Antioxidant*; 6: 27.

Tsai J.H. and Yang J. (2013): Epithelial-mesenchymal plasticity in carcinoma metastasis. *Genes Dev*; 27:2192–206.

Tsai J.-R.,Wang H.-M., Liu P.-L., Chen Y.-H., Yang M.-C., Cho, S.-H., Cheng Y.-J., Yin W.-H., Hwang J.-J. and Chong I.-W. (2012): High expression of heme oxygenase-1 is associated with tumor invasiveness and poor clinical outcome in non-small cell lung cancer patients. *Cell. Oncol. (Dordr.)*; 35: 461–471.

Uno K. *et al.* (2010): Role of Nrf2 in retinal vascular development and the vaso-obliterative phase of oxygen-induced retinopathy. *Exp Eye Res*; 90: 493–500.

Valcarcel-Ares M.N., Gautam T., Warrington J.P., Bailey-Downs L., Sosnowska D., de Cabo R., Losonczy G., Sonntag W.E., Ungvari Z. and Csiszar A. (2012): Disruption of Nrf2 signaling impairs angiogenic capacity of endothelial cells: implications for microvascular aging. *J Gerontol A Biol Sci Med Sci.*

Van Jaarsveld M.T., Helleman J., Boersma A.W., van Kuijk P.F., van Ijcken W.F., Despierre E., Vergote I., Mathijssen R.H., Berns E.M., Verweij J., Pothof J. and Wiemer E.A. (2013): miR-141 regulates KEAP1 and modulates cisplatin sensitivity in ovarian cancer cells. *Oncogene*; 32:4284-4293.

Venugopal R. and Jaiswal A.K. (1996): Nrf1 and Nrf2 positively and c-Fos and Fra1 negatively regulate the human antioxidant response element-mediated expression of NAD(P)H:quinone oxidoreductase1 gene. *Proc Natl Acad Sci USA*; 93:14960–14965.

Vollrath V., Wielandt A.M., Iruretagoyena M., et al. (2006): Role of Nrf2 in the regulation of the Mrp2 (ABCC2) gene. *Biochem J*; 395:599–609.

Wakabayashi, N., Slocum, S.L., Skoko, J.J., Shin, S., Kensler, T.W., 2010. When NRF2talks, who's listening?. *Antiox. Redox. Signal id*; 13 (11): 1649–1663.

Wang J., Zhang M., Zhang L., Cai H., Zhou S., Zhang J. and Wang Y. (2010): Correlation of Nrf2, HO-1, and MRP3 in gallbladder cancer and their relationships to clinicopathologic features and survival. *J Surg Res*; 164:e99–e105.

Wang H., Liu X., Long M., Huang Y., Zhang L., Zhang R., Zheng Y., Liao X., Wang Y., Liao Q., et al. (2016): NRF2 activation by antioxidant antidiabetic agents accelerates tumor metastasis. *Sci. Transl. Med*; 8: 334ra51.

Wang R., An J., Ji F., Jiao H., Sun H. and Zhou D. (2008a): Hypermethylation of theKeap1 gene in human lung cancer cell lines and lung cancer tissues. *Biochem.Biophys. Res. Commun*; 373 (1): 151–154.

Wang X.J., Sun Z., Villeneuve N.F., Zhang S., Zhao F., Li Y., et al. (2008b): Nrf2enhances resistance of cancer cells to chemotherapeutic drugs, the dark side ofNrf2. *Carcinogenesis*; 29 (6): 1235–1243.

World Cancer Report (2014): World Health Organization. 2014. pp. Chapter 1.1.ISBN 9283204298.

Xu X., Zhang Y., Li W., et al. (2014): Wogonin reverses multidrug resistance of human myelogenous leukemia K562/ A02 cells via downregulation of MRP1 expression by inhibiting Nrf2/ARE signaling pathway. *Biochem Pharmacol*; 92:220–234.

You A., Nam C.W., Wakabayashi N., Yamamoto M., Kensler T.W. and Kwak M.K. (2011): Transcription factor Nrf2 maintains the basal expression of Mdm2: An implication of the regulation of p53 signaling by Nrf2. *Arch Biochem Biophys*; 507(2):356-364.

Young L.C., Campling B.G., Cole S.P., et al. (2001): Multidrug resistance proteins MRP3, MRP1, and MRP2 in lung cancer: correlation of protein levels with drug response and messenger RNA levels. *Clin Cancer Res*; 7:1798–1804.

Yuan J.H., Cheng J.Q., Jiang L.Y., et al. (2008): Breast cancer resistance protein expression and 5-fluorouracil resistance. *Biomed Environ Sci*; 21:290–295.

Zhang L., Ding Y., Yuan Z., Liu J., Sun J., Lei F., Wu S., Li S. and Zhang D. (2015): MicroRNA-500 sustains nuclear factor- κ B activation and induces gastric cancer cell proliferation and resistance to apoptosis. *Oncotarget*; 6, 2483–2495.

Zhang M., Zhang C., Zhang L., Yang Q., Zhou S., Wen Q., et al. (2015): Nrf2 is apotential prognostic marker and promotes proliferation and invasion inhuman hepatocellular carcinoma. *BMC Cancer*; 15 (1): 1.

Zhao Y., Hu X., Liu Y., Dong S., Wen Z., He W., Zhang S., Huang Q., and Shi M. (2017): ROS signaling under metabolic stress: cross-talk between AMPK and AKT pathway. *Mol. Cancer*; 16: 79.

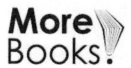
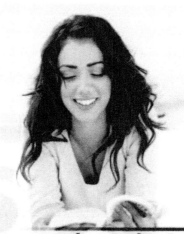 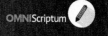

Printed in Great Britain
by Amazon

75036666R00037